Fart Free Vegan

Jon Symons

THANK YOU!

I really appreciate your purchase of my book!
I've created a printable food combining chart as a bonus for this book (since it would be too small to use properly in this book). You can grab a copy here: www.FartFreeVegan.com/chart. I recommend you print it and refer to it while you are reading this book, and when you're planning and preparing your meals.
If you have any questions or comments, contact me at jon@jonsymons.com or at my blog www.JonSymons.com, I'm very happy to hear from you and help out any way I can.

CONTENTS

DISCLAIMER

The information in this book reflects the author's opinions and is not intended to replace medical advice.

Before beginning this or any nutritional program, consult your doctor to be sure it is appropriate for you. If you are unsure of any foods or methods mentioned, you should always defer to your physician's advice.

The author has made every effort to supply accurate information in the creation of this book. The author makes no warranty and accepts no responsibility for any loss or damages arising from the use of the contents of this book.

The reader assumes all responsibility for the use of the information in this text.

INTRODUCTION

Three years ago I was spending 14 to 16 hours a day in bed and had to take a rest break to be able to walk around the block. I had a very serious health condition called Chronic Fatigue Syndrome (CFS).

I had been suffering for over two years and I tried everything to get well again. I had every medical test imaginable, all turned up negative. I had a doctor offer to prescribe antidepressants to me, believing the crushing tiredness was all in my head – it wasn't.

Then, just when I was ready to give up hope, I went to the Hippocrates Health Institute (HHI) in Florida. Besides putting me on a raw vegan diet, I received an amazing education about how the body's immune system and digestive system work.

I learned a lot of important things at HHI, and by implementing that knowledge, my health turned around. I'm writing this book about food combining because I see so many people having trouble getting any results with what should be a very healthy raw or vegan diet. I believe it is primarily due to a lack of knowledge of the digestive system and how the timing and combination of foods can make a huge difference in our energy levels and health.

Even though I am not a scientist, the ideas that I am presenting here are based on proven science. Our bodies are designed to digest food in certain ways and aligning our eating habits with the limitations of our digestive system creates efficient bodies that are healthy and full of energy.

Three years after my first trip to HHI, at age 52, I am healthier than I have ever been in my life. This morning I ran over 2.5 miles, just like I do five times a week. I do yoga or workout with weights three or four times a week as well, but most importantly I am happier than I could have ever imagined was possible. Many people ask me questions about the health recovery that I have made, and I'm sharing this book as the most important and overlooked factor in optimal health (and the easiest to have success with).

When I was sick my immune system was losing a war against all the negative conditions that I had allowed into my system. By eating high-vitality, easily digested raw and living foods, and learning to work with my body's food digesting limitations it freed up energy in my body. That new energy could be applied to fighting illness. My body knew what to do to get better and as soon as I stopped filling it with toxins, while providing my immune system with extra energy to do its job, everything turned around.

I wish the same for you, with whatever health goals you may be pursuing. It's my sincere hope that this book provides you with a step forward in your journey to optimal health and a fantastic life.

SECTION ONE: HOW FOOD COMBINING AFFECTS HEALTH

An Example of a Typical Meal

To get started, I will illustrate the results of poor food combining: putrefaction and fermentation. In my research I discovered a perfect example to illustrate how improper food combining creates gas by showing the digestion process of a typical all-American food - the cheeseburger.

Then I thought, "This is a book for vegans and raw foodies, my readers don't eat stuff like that!" But as I pondered it some more, I realized that almost all of us vegans eat things, from the point of view of food combining, that are just as bad as a cheeseburger, so I decided to do side-by-side examples of the typical cheeseburger and a typical vegan breakfast.

Cheeseburger: bread (starch), beef (protein), cheese (fat) and a slice of tomato (acid fruit). A food combining horror movie!

Typical "healthy" vegan or raw foodie granola breakfast: dehydrated buckwheat cereal (starch), almonds (protein), coconut (fat) and goji or blueberries (acid or fruit). Another food combining horror movie, like a sequel. Imagine a deep announcer voice, "First it was Cheeseburger, now the same award-winning cast, and they've gone vegan - but the plot is just as scary, with all new ingredients."

3

I won't argue that these two meals are equally as harmful in the body (as the burger has a lot more harmful ingredients). However, the stress and difficulty that they create in terms of the digestive process, is nearly identical.

Let's focus on the vegan meal components to demonstrate this.

Breaking it all down, the buckwheat was probably not chewed properly (if you take a look at your stool about 24 – 36 hours after eating your granola, you'll see proof of this as the whole buckwheat kernels exit) and therefore not broken down and mixed with the digestive enzyme in our saliva that is essential for digesting starch. That leads to the buckwheat entering the stomach improperly prepared for further digestion.

The protein in almonds, when detected by the tongue, signals to the stomach to create a high acid environment, which is necessary to break down and digest protein.

Unfortunately the high acid content that is required in the stomach to process the almonds, almost completely stops the digestion of the buckwheat starch, as the enzyme that digests starch requires a neutral or alkaline (not acidic) environment. This results in the buckwheat starch exiting the stomach undigested and this leads to it eventually becoming food for gas producing bacteria further down the digestive tract.

Then the fats from the coconut slow down the digestive process as they take longer to break down in the stomach than either proteins or starches. Fats also don't do well in an acidic environment which was created for the protein, so they, just like the starchy buckwheat, will not be properly digested when they do leave the stomach.

Lastly, the fruits are acidic, so they also inhibit the digestion of the starchy buckwheat, but the worst thing about the fruit is that they are digested very quickly. Because of their high water content, fruits would normally spend very little time in the stomach, but when they are mixed in the same mouthful or meal as protein, carbs or fat, they cannot move out of the stomach until the rest of the foods they entered with have been processed; the slowest food determines the transit time in the stomach, to the detriment of any faster foods that are in the mixture.

Instead of moving quickly down the digestive tract as it was meant to, the fruit begins to ferment, giving off toxic and foul smelling gas, which if chronic, leads to health problems.

In a single bite of this meal there are at least four different digestive challenges for our body, that require completely different digestive times, different enzymes and different acidity levels at various stages of the process. Our body is a magnificent machine that can handle all of these circumstances, but it simply doesn't possess the tools to handle them all at once.

Unfortunately, the best we can hope for in this meal is very slow digestion of the entire mess which will result in fermentation. In the worst case scenario, digestion is never completed and the partially digested foods are pushed through our entire system slowly releasing poisons as the bacteria feed on the undigested pieces. In either case, the result is a very tiny bit of self poisoning as the gas and other waste products are absorbed back into our blood stream and organs.

Of course, this is just one meal and our body is strong and adaptable, but if we multiply the effects of this meal by hundreds or even thousands of overly complex meals, over time, the effect on our health can be significantly negative.

The Concept of Food Combining

The basis of food combining is an understanding of the chemical and physical processes that make up our digestive system. While what we eat is certainly a key to our health, how the food we eat gets digested and what gets extracted as nutrients is equally essential to our physical well being. Our digestive system has very real limitations that affect the extraction of energy and nourishment from our food.

Correct food combining works with the enzymes and gastric juices in our body to create an efficient and effective process of digestion. Improper food combining impedes and in some cases prevents the digestion of foods. This can result in fermentation in the intestines and uncomfortable pressure, gas and irritation.

In the long term this digestive irritation can lead to health issues ranging from allergies to more serious conditions that weaken the immune system. Removal of these irritating digestive disruptions by proper food combining can result in significant improvements in many health symptoms.

In short, our health begins in our gut. When we learn to be in harmony with our digestive system, better health and proper weight will follow.

What is a Fart?

Before the days of electronic gas detectors, underground coal miners would carry caged canaries down into the mine shafts with them. If dangerous gases like carbon monoxide or methane leaked into the mine, they would kill the bird before killing the miners, providing a warning to leave the mine immediately.

Chronic gassiness in the form of farts or burps or even irregular stools is a warning sign that things are not right in our body. Since our bodies are so amazingly talented at adaptation and death avoidance, we are most likely not in imminent danger, but if these symptoms are present on a regular basis, many unpleasant health concerns will not be far behind.

The average person will pass gas about thirteen times a day producing a total of about two cups of flatus, as it is called when emitted from the rectum.

What Causes Gas in Our Digestive System?

Farts are caused by gas that is created by three things: air that is swallowed when we eat, normal chemical reactions in our digestive systems and bacterial fermentation of undigested foods.

The gas that is swallowed from the air contains nitrogen and oxygen. It is completely normal and our body releases this air as a harmless fart or a burp.

In the duodenum (the part in our digestive system between the stomach and small intestine) we form carbon dioxide gas by a chemical reaction of hydrochloric acid from the stomach with the bicarbonate of the pancreatic secretions. This reaction, which produces small amounts of odorless gas is also normal.

The third type of gas production is primarily methane and hydrogen sulfide which is formed through bacterial fermentation in the small intestine and colon. These gases are formed when bacteria act on undigested food. How undigested foods get into the colon and small intestine is what we are going to discover and learn to change in this book.

There are foods that are naturally more difficult to digest. These include: cauliflower, Brussels sprouts, legumes (peas, beans, lentils), broccoli, cabbage, dried and sulfured fruits, cucumbers, celery, apples, carrots, onions, garlic, cantaloupe, radishes, grapes, raisins, and under ripe bananas.

Even though these foods are a challenge, it is not the foods that are really the problem. The problem is that we are ignorant of the limitations of our digestive systems, so we eat foods in a way that they cannot be digested. Our digestive system developed when our lives were a lot simpler. There just weren't any buffets, four course meals, or drive through fast food joints 100,000 years ago.

Other causes of gas and indigestion are like a who's who list of unhealthy foods: caffeine, alcohol, salt, refined sugar and processed oils all serve as difficult-to-digest irritants. Also there are nutritional deficiencies of digestive enzymes, hydrochloric acid and B vitamins which can be factors in digestive problems.

Food allergies or sensitivities may also result in excessive gas production as can too much vitamin C or vitamin C-rich foods such as oranges.

In this book we are going to focus on the other *major* cause of indigestion (from here on, I'll use the word indigestion rather than fart, because it is more accurate) which is not eating in alliance with the limitations of our digestive system. This shows up as the way we eat, primarily not chewing our food properly and the way we combine foods in meals that creates mixtures in our stomach that are impossible to digest.

Once you learn some very simple rules you'll be amazed at the difference in comfort that you will experience in your digestive system. For some reason this knowledge is not common, but it is very straightforward and the benefits of following these simple guidelines can be profound.

Putrification and Fermentation

"Decomposition or rotting, the breakdown of organic matter usually by bacterial action, resulting in the formation of other substances of less complex constitution with the evolution of ammonia or its derivatives and hydrogen sulfide; characterized usually by the presence of toxic or malodorous products."

The definition of "putrification" from medical-dictionary.thefreedictionary.com

In short, putrification is a result of decomposition, as opposed to digestion, of protein by microorganisms which produces foul smelling and toxic by-products.

Fermentation is the decomposition of sugars and starches by microorganisms into carbon dioxide, acid and alcohol. Digestion reduces food down to a smaller and useful solution without damaging its organic qualities, whereas fermentation simply destroys the food and creates toxins.

Fart Free for Weight Loss

How does proper food combining lead to weight loss and maintaining an ideal weight? It's simple: get in harmony with your body, and it will reward you with its perfect weight.

Since weight loss is one of the health benefits that many are after when they choose a vegan diet it is worth mentioning here that fat in the body is created by the metabolism of excess carbohydrates in the body. This is why a raw food diet, when done correctly, will lead the body to its ideal weight; because there are not excess carbs coming into the body, so there isn't a possibility of fat storage that leads to weight gain.

Excess carbs doesn't only mean eating too much rice or potato. Any starches (including fruits or starchy vegetables) that are improperly combined and eaten with protein can lead to our body storing these carbs as fats.

The primary benefit of food combining is that it frees up energy as the digestive system becomes more efficient. Our body will use this new energy for all manner of repairs including detoxification, healing and weight normalization.

The other major weight loss benefit of understanding food combining is emotionally. Most people, myself included, have developed a habit of emotional eating; we eat not only when we are hungry, but we eat when we want to feel better.

We've all seen a parent with a screaming child at the supermarket stuff a candy into the kid's mouth to shut it up. This creates an association in the child that when it is feeling bad a sugary treat can be used to change their mood. Most of us learned this type of eating as kids. Combine this with the addictive nature of processed sugary and high fat foods and it's a recipe for abusive emotionally-based eating.

This certainly was my story. Although I didn't gain that much weight, my body developed illnesses as a result of my addictive eating.

This book can help with weight loss by increasing your awareness of how you eat and the effects this has on your body. Not only will you learn what to do to create a more efficient digestive system which will naturally lead to your body releasing stored fats and toxins, but also, being more conscious of your eating will have a profound effect on many aspects of your relationship to your body.

These days I am more aware of why I'm eating and when I'm eating in an addictive manner (which is when I am most likely to choose a meal that is a poorly combined mess of ingredients). With awareness I'm able to stop myself and say, this isn't really what I want to do. This is also where self love comes into the picture.

Self love is the ability to, as an adult, re-parent ourselves. Instead of acting out the old patterns we learned of eating to adjust our emotions, we can be like a loving parent towards ourselves and gently guide our eating choices into a more healthy direction.

We can take that child from the supermarket, that is still inside of all of us, and validate its (our) feelings so that we no longer need to eat to cover them up, or stuff them down. Then we will be free from emotional eating and we can make better choices in our diet.

These healthy choices are ones that serve us better in the long term and help us let go of needing short term gratification from food.

Common Digestive Health Problems

Our gut has a lot of bacteria living it. To overly simplify, there are good guys and bad guys. The good guys are the ones we hear about in the TV commercials these days; selling acidophilus and bifidobacterium have become big business because people have abused their digestive systems and the good guys are in short supply in a lot of people's guts.

Then there are the bad guys like e-coli, salmonella, staphylococcus and others, not to mention parasites, fungi and yeast like Candida.

Even the so-called bad guys are not really that bad. In a healthy body the good guys and bad guys exist in kind of stalemate. The good bacteria are like a police force that keeps the unpleasant bacteria under control.

Having the undesirable bacteria, yeast and parasites in control of regions of the digestive system can lead to all manner of unpleasant symptoms: gas, bloating, cramps, diarrhea, constipation, allergies and fatigue, just for a start. If any of these become chronic they can lead to more serious conditions such as leaky gut syndrome, Crohn's disease, irritable bowel syndrome and others including a compromised immune system.

There are many things we can do to aid our immune system and the good healthy bacteria in keeping our digestive flora balanced. They include avoiding sugars, getting plenty of rest, and exercise. Then of course, there is proper food combining, which starves the bad bacteria by cutting off their food supply.

Chewing properly and eating in harmonious combinations reduces the amount of undigested food that is travelling in the gastrointestinal (GI) tract. These undigested pieces actually feed the nasty bacteria which cannot thrive without an ample source of food.

The other thing that proper combining achieves is that it maintains an optimal pH level in the GI tract. An acidic environment, often from too much undigested protein, is the ideal place for the bad bacteria to thrive, whereas healthy bacteria require a neutral or slightly alkaline environment.

In the rest of this book I'll go into more detail about what is happening in our digestive system and why we need to simplify and streamline our eating.

Along the way we'll bust a few more supposedly healthy vegan and raw food habits, just like the granola meal example above. Then we'll provide some simple guidelines for a harmonious and blissful belly while still enjoying the yummy foods

SECTION TWO: THE TYPES OF FOOD AND WHY WE EAT THEM

Why We Eat

Take a moment here and think back to your last meal and ask yourself, "why did I eat?"

If you're like most people there will be one or more of many reasons; "I was hungry", "I always eat dinner at 6pm", "I was out for a meal with friends", etc.

Why we eat is a question that most people never consider. We just do it because our stomach starts to feel uncomfortable if we don't put stuff into it every few hours.

But why we eat is a question that is worth some consideration, especially for seekers of optimal health or weight loss.

The real answer is that food provides energy and nutrients that our body can then use to create and sustain our tissues, bones, organs, blood, muscles, skin etc. Nutrients in foods are compounds in the food that can be extracted and used by the body. These include the chemical compounds we are all probably familiar with: carbs, fats, proteins, vitamins and minerals and fiber or cellulose.

The point here is that all food must be processed by the digestive system to be useful to our body. The digestive system allows the food to be broken down into the components that the body can then use as ingredients and resources for all the other systems that need to be created and maintained for us to go on living.

Our job, as we strive to be healthy, is to understand the needs of our body and the resources available within our body to extract nourishment. Then it is up to us to provide the proper foods, in the correct combinations to allow our digestive system to function well and provide us with vibrant health.

The next step in understanding our digestive system and how it works is to take a closer look at the different types of foods.

Types of Food

The cornerstone of understanding our digestive system and how to align our food combining with our body is to get clear about the types of foods we are eating. Our body has different methods to process different foods and food classifications have been created to help us align our eating with our body's digestive methods.

The first thing to realize about the food types and classifications is that they are generalizations. No one food is 100% protein or 100% starch, even though this is what we are led to believe by the food marketing and diet industry.

All foods have a measure of protein in them, but some are also quite starchy. Beans for example are thought of as a protein food by many vegans and vegetarians, but they are more correctly classified as a starchy protein and placed in the starch or carbohydrate category when it comes to the rules of proper food combining.

Another big fallacy with regard to food types is that protein only comes from certain foods: i.e. meats, or for us vegans and raw foodies, nuts and seeds. This is far from the truth.

As a raw vegan, I am often asked, where I get my protein from. The answer I've come up with is to say, the same place that a race horse gets it: from leafy greens. Not only do greens (especially raw, living greens like sunflower and pea sprouts) contain large amounts of protein, but they also provide the protein in a form that is much easier for the body to extract and make use of.

However, for the purpose of this food combining book, we will stick to the traditional food classifications because getting this straightened out in our eating is what will make the biggest difference in our digestive efficiency.

NOTE: in case you missed it at the beginning of this book, I prepared a free printable chart of the types of foods and the food combining rules, which you can grab from my website:

http://www.fartfreevegan.com/chart

Protein

What's the first thing you think of when the word "protein" comes into your mind? For me and I'm betting the majority of people, it's energy! For a few more enlightened folks, mostly gym rats, the answer maybe muscle – which is a lot closer to the truth.

The truth is, protein is not required, at all, as an energy source in our body. We use protein only for growth (an example would be a body builder who is creating or growing new muscle) and tissue repair and replacement. A mother feeds her baby breast milk, a high quality protein. The baby is in a rapid growth phase and having a sufficient supply of protein in an easily digestible form is essential.

We all need protein, but the idea that if you're fatigued or weak that you are lacking protein is far from true.

Protein is not needed for increased energy, as a source of fuel or muscle energy. Our body can produce fuel from protein, but it does it by breaking the protein down into carbohydrates, which is a very energy intensive process, and it only does this when there aren't any other carbohydrates available.

Good quality vegan sources of protein include: seeds like hemp, sesame, flax, sunflower and pumpkin. Nuts like walnuts, pine nuts, pecans and almonds. The highest quality proteins on the planet are chlorella and spirulina.

As mentioned above, many foods that are not thought of as protein do in fact contain significant amounts of proteins. Coconut, dried fruits, avocados, bananas, Brussels sprouts, broccoli and romaine lettuce are some examples.

Not that I recommend eating them, but for the sake of clarity, I'll mention that animal products are also considered high-protein foods.

Carbohydrates and Starches

There is so much attention to proteins in our modern media, but it is starches that are by far the most important type of food for humans. Everything that we do, whether it's thinking, writing this book, reading, walking, talking, breathing and even digesting, is powered by starches or carbs being converted into glucose to be burned as energy by our body.

Human beings are "carbon-based" and the word "carbs" is a nickname for carbon containing compounds that we require as food energy.

Getting into a discussion about the pros and cons of popular low-carb diets is beyond the scope of this book. But one thing is certain: if your body doesn't have carbs to burn as fuel, you will not be able to function, so what diet you're on is not going to matter!

For a vegan, high quality carbs include grains (best eaten sprouted, while avoiding the ones with gluten), sprouted and/or cooked beans and soy. I added soy in here because it is correctly classified as a carb and popular as a vegetarian and vegan food, however it has usually been hybridized and genetically modified so heavily that it is very difficult to digest in its own right. Personally, for this reason I avoid soy completely in my diet.

Also in the carbs category are starchy vegetables like winter squash, potatoes and corn. Then there are some less starchy vegetables in this category: carrots, beets, and peas and beans in the pod.

Another excellent source of carbohydrates is fruits. Sweet fresh fruits are high in water content, very easy to digest and high in natural sugars, which is what the body actually converts starches into to create fuel.

But before you gorge yourself on fruits thinking you'll have endless energy, remember that fruits are great but they have some very important food combining considerations that we'll learn in the next couple of sections.

Fruits

Fruits provide us with a very healthy energy source and minerals and nutrients that are essential and cannot be found in other foods. Understanding fruit and how our body digests them is very important as they are a major cause of indigestion due to a lack of proper food combining when eating them.

The typical vegan diet abuses fruits badly, and one of my reasons for writing this book was to help people who are struggling with vegan and raw food diets primarily because of not knowing how to eat fruits properly. Once we understand how our body digests fruits, we can combine them in ways that respect our body's processes, and get the benefits of these amazing foods without the indigestion.

For the purposes of food combining classification there are four subcategories of fruit. They each have some slight differences and if you reflect on the fruits found in each category, you'll develop an intuitive sense of what the differences are.

Sweet Fruits

These include bananas, and dried fruits like figs, dates and raisins.

Subacid Fruits

This category contains most of our common fruits: apples, less traditional grape varieties, peaches, cherries, blueberries (and most other berries), mangoes, pears and kiwi

Acid Fruits

Include citrus like oranges, grapefruits, lemons and also strawberries, pomegranates and pineapple.

Melons

Watermelon, cantaloupe and others are a special category of fruit for the purpose of digestion. They are the quickest food to digest; therefore they must be eaten alone and on an empty stomach. We'll go into this in more detail in the next section.

The other important rule about fruit is that they must be eaten ripe to be considered a fruit. A banana that is not ripe is much starchier than a ripe one. It can be difficult to find quality fruit in our modern world, when fruit is picked three weeks before it is ripe and transported 2000 miles or more to our store!

Consider our ancestors who ate one type of fruit at a time as it dropped from a tree. This was the type of fruit eating experience that our digestive system was developed for, and the closer we can come to eating in that manner, the better our digestive health will be.

Fats

Something that is not well understood is that plants contain fats. Olive oil and sunflower oil are oils that are extracted from plants.

The beauty is that once you remove animal products and processed foods from your diet, you will be getting fats in perfect proportion from the original sources... as long as you don't overdo it on oils.

Fats are very seldom eaten alone, especially on a raw or vegan diet. The only real source of concentrated fat is found in oils (olive, hemp, sunflower etc). In my own diet I treat these as processed foods, which they are, and use them very sparingly. If you are eating a healthy vegan or raw diet with a variety of foods, you should not need to even think about fats as you will automatically be getting just the right amount from the natural fat content of your food.

Three other non-concentrated, sources of fat in a healthy vegan or raw diet are avocados, coconut and nuts (sprouted and dehydrated below 105 degrees F.). Most nuts contain about 10 - 20 percent protein and about 50 - 70 percent fat.

I mentioned it earlier but fat intake does not lead to fat storage in the body. Excess carbs or starch in the diet lead to metabolized storage of fats or weight gain. Intake of excess fats can cause other problems such as strain on the liver or gall bladder.

About once every few months I will eat a bit of cooked food. I use coconut oil for cooking, as I believe it is the oil that is least damaged and harmful to use when heated, which is why I mention it here.

To summarize our discussion of fats: use fatty foods sparingly and use concentrated fats *very* sparingly.

If you notice that you have particularly difficult time digesting fats, then try eating some bitter greens like arugula or dandelion greens before the rest of your meal (or try "bitters" herbal formulas). The bitter taste, which is all but forgotten in our modern diet, actually stimulates the liver to produce more bile which is essential in the digestion of fats.

Vegetables

Fresh raw vegetables should be the cornerstone of every diet. This is especially true for leafy green vegetables that contain protein, carbs, fats and minerals in a form that our body can easily absorb. We all intuitively know this, but not that many people actually follow their own wisdom.

For raw or vegan diets non starchy vegetables can be our primary foods. They include leafy greens, sprouts like sunflower or peas or alfalfa, lettuce, celery, summer squash like zucchini, kale and chard.

In food combining, the non-starchy vegetables are the most versatile foods. They can be combined with the most variety of other foods, and can still be digested properly.

A sub group of the vegetables is starchy vegetables that include: beans, beets, carrots, corn, peas, white potatoes, yams or sweet potatoes and winter squash. These vegetables have much higher starch content than the vegetables above, and will be treated as carbs when planning meals that follow proper food combining rules presented later in the forth chapter of this book.

Later in this book I have a section on fiber and will get into it in detail, but I'll mention here that kale and broccoli are two high fiber vegetables that when eaten raw, can cause indigestion, even when combined correctly. Over time your body will handle these foods without issue, but in the beginning, making smoothies with your kale and broccoli can help break down the fiber which is the cause of the problem.

Special Case Foods

Tomatoes

Tomatoes are actually a subacid fruit but they don't have the sugar content of other fruits. Traditionally they are used as a vegetable, which presents digestive issues. Tomatoes, like most fruits, do not combine well with most other foods, especially starches as the acid content interferes with starch digestion.

Personally I only eat tomatoes alone on an empty stomach, but they will combine with a leafy green salad, as long as you eat the salad before any other foods.

Avocados

Avocados are a fruit that is a combination fat/protein food. They can, depending on variety have up to 2% protein, which is more than milk for example, and they contain upwards of 15% fat. They also have a high amount of fiber.

Avocados, due to their fat content, slow down the digestive system. This makes avocados a poor choice with other fruits – including tomatoes.

The best way to eat an avocado is as part of a salad meal.

Coconut

Coconut is obviously a nut, although an unusual one that we typically eat as liquid. The rest of the coconut is the meat, and this part of the coconut is a protein source but is also high in fat.

Coconut meat should be eaten in limited quantities, is best combined with leafy green vegetables, and should not be mixed with fruits as the fat content slows down digestion and will cause fermentation.

Coconut has a lot of amazing qualities, and there are entire books dedicated to how to get the health benefits from coconut, but I want to share a few hard-earned words of caution from my own research and experience.

The white coconuts still in their husks that you find at the grocery store are a great way to have "fresh" young coconut even if you don't live in a tropical climate. But, coconuts do not have white husks, they are brown. Those ones you are buying have been bleached and or dipped in formaldehyde as a preservative.

Be very careful or use gloves when handling them, and if when you open them and the liquid is even slightly pink, don't drink it, it means the formaldehyde has soaked into the nut and contaminated the coconut juice.

The next consideration is about dried coconut meat. See if you can find "raw" which is packaged just like other coconut meat, but it has been dried at lower than 110 degrees Fahrenheit which preserves the enzymes and a lot of the amazing nutrients in the coconut. You'll get a lot more nutrition from eating coconut that is still raw.

Lastly is coconut oil, which is oh so yummy. But as I have mentioned earlier oils are a concentrated form of food, so they are hard to digest. Use coconut oil very sparingly. Concentrated foods, especially fats, can be addictive, so be very aware when you are using it, if you start to crave more and more, put it aside.

Olives

Olives are also a fruit that is high in fat. Olives, as most of us consume them, are far from a healthy food, as they are processed and mixed with salt and preservatives. Natural, sundried olives are acceptable. Olive oil is concentrated and should therefore be used in very limited quantities as it can be difficult to digest.

A side note about olive oil: it is very rare to find high quality olive oil in a regular grocery or even health food store. Real extra virgin cold pressed olive oil tastes very different than what is typically used. It also has a "Picked on" date and a "Pressed On" date. Quality oil will always have these dates on it, and it must be consumed within two years.

The health benefits attributed to olive oil are found in this type of quality oil and not the dead and over processed oils that you have likely been using (even if you are buying certified organic, first cold pressed extra virgin). I've listed an example in my resources page:

FartFreeVegan.com/I-use

Juices and Smoothies

Juices and smoothies are near and dear to almost every vegan and raw foodie. They are quick and easy, transportable, easy to digest and extremely healthy, right?

Yes and no.

Unfortunately there are some simple rules with juices and smoothies that are often broken, and these can undermine all the benefits of liquid foods.

We'll talk more about this one later, but fruits do not mix with any vegetables except leafy greens and celery. This simple rule is broken very often as people add fruits to their juices and smoothies to improve taste or add sweetness, but unfortunately gas or indigestion often follows and the benefits of the juices are lost.

Now that we have that sacred cow out of the way, and we assume you will be having your juices with only vegetables (or an all-fruit juice or smoothie is okay) let's see what other guidelines can help us derive the maximum nutrients out of our liquid foods.

Juices and smoothies are not the same. While they could have exactly the same ingredients; for me a typical juice is sunflower sprouts, pea sprouts, cucumber and celery, a juice is made using a juicer (I use only a slow-speed masticating juicer) which extracts juice from the vegetables and removes the fiber. A smoothie on the other hand is made in a blender and simply liquefies the ingredients and is diluted with water.

While juice and smoothie might have the same ingredients and look almost identical, in our digestive system they are treated quite differently.

Because the fiber is removed, juice can pass almost directly through the stomach and into the small intestine making it very easy on the digestive system. Close to 95% of the nutrients in juice can be harvested making it an extremely efficient and highly dense way to supply nourishment to the body. Juice made with high quality organic greens is the healthiest food I can put in my body. I make 20 to 30 ounces a day and have been doing it for three years and have seen a huge difference in my health because of it.

A smoothie on the other hand, is really still a solid food (since none of the fiber has been removed) that is diluted and liquefied. It still needs to be digested in the same way that any other solid food does. The advantage of a smoothie is that the food has been broken down; the chewing has been done so the body will have an easier time breaking the food down in the initial stages of digestion.

However, smoothies are not as efficient or effective at supplying nourishment as juices as our body still must deal with the fiber by extracting it from the liquid, a digestive step that is not required with juices.

Chew Your Juice!

As we wrap up our discussion of juices and smoothies there is one other important point about liquid foods: they still have to be "chewed!"

Sounds weird, I know, but as we'll learn a bit later, chewing plays the role of not only breaking down the food into tiny bits, but also in mixing it with our saliva which contains enzymes that are essential for the effective digestion of any food, including juices.

So don't forget to chew your juices and smoothies, if you just chug it, you'll be missing the majority of the benefits of what is probably the best possible food you can put in your body.

Coffee and Tea

These drinks have an interesting and profound effect on the digestive system. Many people drink coffee and teas for their "pick me up" energy boost, but there is also another known and popular side effect of these drinks: they have a laxative effect. To the many people who suffer from the very unpleasant symptom of constipation, any relief is appreciated.

However, the reason that coffee and tea are laxatives is not good news for our digestive system. These drinks, due to their acidity, cause the stomach to release food pre-maturely (undigested).

Food then enters the small intestine before the processes in the stomach have been completed properly and poor absorption of nutrients and fermentation are the results.

Summary of the Types of Foods

Now that we understand what we need to eat to properly nourish and energize our body, and we have categorized the various foods, we are ready for the next step which is to take a look at the processes and chemicals in our digestive system and how they do their work.

We will see how the types of food categories are treated differently by the body and from this we will begin to get an understanding of why food combining has such a big effect on our well being.

SECTION THREE: THE DIGESTIVE SYSTEM

A Chemical & Mechanical Factory

The next step in our path to perfect digestion is to understand a little bit about the chemical process of the body and how they break down our food. Have no fear, this isn't science class, but I always find that knowing a little bit of detail helps create a more vivid and complete picture of what is going on, which helps to motivate the changes and inspire us to use healthier combinations.

The digestive system involves a long chain of actions and reactions that actually begins before food enters our body, and ends with the waste products being deposited into a toilet bowl.

The digestive process has been studied extensively and the chemical reactions that break down our food in an efficient and effective manner are well documented. Given this fact, it is surprising that so little attention is paid to the rules of our own bodies when it comes to digesting food. I can only guess that in general people dislike change so intensely, that they would rather continue to travel the well beaten path rather than make adjustments to their diets (for example the hamburger is a classic food combining no-no due to the presence of both protein and carbs in the same meal) which would lead to improved health.

But thankfully you're reading this book and you can make the change to being a more aware eater, and becoming an indigestion-free vegan!

Let's get started by looking at the primary component of our digestive system: enzymes.

Enzymes and Gastric Juices

In order to receive nutrients from our food, which are in general quite complex structures, and use them to benefit the body, the foods we eat need to be broken down into much simpler compounds.

Enzymes are present in all living things. They facilitate transformations of every kind. An example of this process is when you cut open an apple; it is a type of enzyme that is released in the apple that turns it brown due to oxidization. What is happening is the apple is beginning to decay and break down; just as the food in our stomachs breaks down as the enzymes begin to act upon it.

There are many different types of enzymes and in the next section we will explore the main ones in some detail. The most important thing to realize about enzymes is that each enzyme has a very specific task and is only effective for one type of food category (remember the previous section of food types).

Enzymes are like tools. When you want to drive a screw into a piece of wood, if you try and do it with a wrench, your results will be very poor. The enzymes used for digesting proteins are almost completely ineffective for digesting carbs.

Imagine a tree that has fallen in the forest. Over enough time, bacteria will decompose the tree back into soil which can then be used by the forest as nutrients to grow a new tree. But bacteria is slow, it takes many years to process the tree and it produces gases which are not a problem in the forest, but have nowhere to go in our digestive tract. Enzymes are catalysts that speed up chemical reactions, like the digestion of food.

Each enzyme only acts on one type or category of food or one product of previous enzyme activity. And each enzyme functions only at a certain pH level.

Let's take a brief step back to science class. All we need to know about pH is that some substances are acidic and low pH (hydrochloric acid that is found in our stomach, vinegar, acetic acid in fruits, and carbonic acid that is found in soft drinks) and some are alkaline which are high on the pH scale (bleach, ammonia, baking soda).

Directly in the middle of the pH scale, is pure water, which is neutral: neither acidic nor alkaline.

Our stomach is typically an acidic environment, which is necessary for the digestion of protein and to kill potential parasites and bad bacteria in our food. From there the rest of our digestive system becomes more and more alkaline which is the perfect environment for enzyme digestion of other types of food and for healthy bacteria to operate in the small and large intestines.

In summary, enzymes are catalysts that help our digestive system break down food into more useful, less complex pieces. Also we learned that each food category has only one type of enzyme that is effective in breaking it down. And each enzyme functions only in one specific pH level environment in the body.

As we build our picture of proper food digestion we now see that our body is a simple system that has some very specific requirements to work optimally.

The only other factor we need to put it all together is timing and sequencing. Like an auto assembly line (the digestive system is more like a dis-assembly line where the food is taken apart and made into smaller and smaller pieces) if the car parts are not lined up with the correct tools at the time when that tool needs to do its job, the system breaks. If the car passes by the door painting machine, but the trim and window are already on the door, a mess is going to be the result.

Our digestive system functions in the same way. Each step impacts the next one's effectiveness.

Next we'll take a look at how the body releases these enzymes and why timing of foods entering the system, which is what food combining really boils down to, is so important for perfect digestion.

Peristalsis – the Body's Assembly Line

Peristalsis is not an actual part of our digestive system, but rather a process that is very important. Peristalsis is a sequential series of muscle movements that move food through the digestive system like a conveyor belt moves parts through an assembly line.

The first step is swallowing your food. The food slides down your esophagus and into your stomach via a sequential tightening of the muscles in your esophagus to push the food lower and lower.

Peristalsis moves food from mouth, to stomach to small intestine to the colon and then into your toilet. But there is one other important peristalsis action; it agitates food in your stomach. The muscles around your stomach contort in an effort to shake the stomach to aid in the breakdown of food by the digestive enzymes.

Think of your stomach like a washing machine and the enzymes are the detergent. The washing machine agitates to separate the dirt from the clothes in the same way the stomach peristalsis agitates the food particles to break them down into smaller and more absorbable particles.

The reason this is important in our desire to be indigestion free is to understand the limitations of the body. Imagine we want to make a smoothie, so we toss a bunch of ingredients into a blender, flick it on, and voila, we have a nice liquid smoothie.

Our digestive system has the same goal with the food we eat; to turn it into the consistency of a smoothie so the nutrients can be extracted. But there are no electric motors or ultra sharp cutting blades available to our stomach.

The larger, and more complex the individual pieces of food are and the more complex the combination of food is, the more difficult it is for the digestive system to break it down into a useful liquid.

Fiber & Cellulose

Fiber is not really a type of food, but it deserves a short introduction in this book because of its importance in our health and the effect it has on our digestion.

There are some medical researchers who claim that lack of fiber in the diet is a contributing factor to almost all disease. The typical North American diet is woefully lacking in fiber. Processed and fast foods do not contain the fiber necessary for proper digestion. But it's debatable whether or not it's the lack of fiber or the lack of nutrition in that diet that causes problems.

Luckily a well balanced vegan diet (one that includes a vast majority of raw foods) does have amble fiber and nutrients. Fiber is the indigestible part of food and it moves through the system without being broken down and is expelled in our stool.

Foods that are high in fiber are more work for our digestive system. Most of us who were raised on a typical diet with few raw vegetables have digestive systems that have the muscle tone of a couch potato!

When we start to eat a high-fiber diet of lots of raw veggies, it is like taking Mr. Couch Potato (i.e. our digestive system) and sending it straight to the fitness club for a two-hour workout on the stair machine – it's going to suffer.

The digestive system, as we learned above is a series of muscles, and high-fiber foods require more muscular effort to break down.

It is for this reason that someone who is new to raw food may have some indigestion even if they follow proper food combining rules. This is only a temporary state while their digestive system is building new muscle strength and being transformed into a lean, mean digestive machine from the workout provided by those raw veggies.

Many people just starting on a raw diet use smoothies and blend their vegetables to give the body a head start on breaking down the fiber. Just be aware that over-blending raw food can lead to oxidation and the destruction of enzymes in the food, so blend as little as possible.

In general I'm not a big fan of supplements, but when I first started on my raw food diet, I used digestive enzymes to ease my transition and help my digestive system until it had the strength to properly digest my high-fiber diet on its own. In the recommended resources section at the end of this book, I have linked to my favorite enzymes.

A Tour of Our Digestive System in Action

The first phase of the digestive process begins before food comes anywhere near our fork. Thinking about something yummy to eat or seeing something tasty actually puts the digestive system into action. The saliva glands in the mouth begin to produce enzymes to prepare for food entering to be broken down once chewing begins, and the gastric juices in the stomach are readied for action.

Now we know why TV commercials of addictive junk foods and fast food burgers are so effective, we are trained to have a physical response to this stimulation, and once those digestive system juices are flowing in the body, it is almost instinctive for us to satisfy those digestive system cravings.

In the following tour of the digestive system we will see what happens to food once it enters our body; the process of being broken down by our digestive system into nutrients that we can then use for growth, repair and energy.

The entire process of digestion can be summarized by one goal: to break large complex pieces of food into smaller and simpler pieces that can be used to create energy and to grow and repair tissues.

Imagine a home that was filled with beautiful and useful fixtures and building materials, but the home itself was no longer desirable. Workers could come in, dismantle the parts of the home, and break all the pieces down into planks (like hardwood flooring) or architectural moldings, and stained glass windows. Then set those valuable pieces aside to be used in a new home, and send the rest of the useless pieces like old rotten roof shingles, off to the dump.

Our digestive system works the same way, trying to recycle our food into useful pieces. Obviously then, what foods and how we put them into our system makes a very big difference in the kinds of materials that our body has at its disposal to build and maintain our bodies.

Our Mouth

The first step in our digestive process is the mouth. I remember when I was a kid, my grandmother would tell me, "Chew each bite of food 32 times!"

I would start to count, chewing on each count, and oh my god, 32 was a heck of lot of chewing. Eating a meal would have taken three hours. But Grandma's crazy rule was well based in digestive science.

The mouth is arguably the most underappreciated part of the digestive system. Watch most people eat and you would think that the mouth is not much more important that the top of a funnel to stuff food into the throat and provide a little bit of titillation via the taste buds.

The act of chewing food properly is probably the most important step in the digestive process. After food leaves our mouth, all the body has to break it down into useful nutrients are chemicals, enzymes and bacteria and a little bit of muscle movement to swish things around.

When food is properly chewed, the rest of the process is many orders of magnitude more efficient. When a huge piece of food, especially a more complex or poorly combined mouthful, enters the stomach, vast amounts of resources are used to try and break the food down into a liquid form which is where the digestive enzymes need it to be before they can begin their process.

Chewing

Here are a couple of sayings (that didn't come from my Grandmother) that I use to help reinforce the idea of properly chewing:

"Drink your food and chew your juice."

This saying, which I learned at Hippocrates, points out that food needs to be liquefied to be properly digested, and even juice needs to be mixed with the enzymes in our saliva to be effectively processed.

And:

"You don't have teeth in your stomach."

This is an obvious statement that makes the point that your mouth is the only chance your body has to liquefy its food.

The process is like a conveyer belt, if big pieces come in, likely they are not processed properly by the stomach in time, and then they are passed on to the small intestine in a form that will make it very difficult for the small intestine to properly do its job, and so it goes through the system.

It only happens once in a while, this doesn't present a big problem as our body is amazingly flexible, but years and years of stress being placed on the entire digestive system by having to attempt to compensate for unchewed food, can lead to many health symptoms.

Saliva

The other reason chewing is very important is that our saliva contains an enzyme that is essential in the digestion of starchy foods. While we are chewing our food, we are mixing it with our saliva and the digestive process is officially started.

The Taste Buds

The last function of the mouth in the digestive system involves the taste buds. Our taste buds actually signal to the rest of the system what types of foods are coming in, and our body prepares the digestive juices and enzymes that are most appropriate for the digestion of those foods. As we will see in some detail, our body treats all the categories of food differently; it uses different tools for the digestion of each type of food.

There are really only two things about our digestion that we control: the first is what foods we put into our body, and the second is how well we chew what does come into our body.

The mouth gives us a very interesting clue about the need to eat a simple diet. Our body uses different enzymes and other digestive juices to process the different food types. The mouth signals the brain to release these tools based on what is tasted in the mouth, but the food we typically eat is so complex that we are constantly signally our digestive system, "be ready for everything, all at once."

The Tongue

In yoga, yogis believe that every living thing has Prana, or life force energy. Chewing food liberates the Prana energy from the food, which is absorbed into, and is added to, our life force energy through our tongue. This energy is like the spiritual nutrition of what we are eating, as opposed to the physical nutrition which is extracted by the rest of our digestive system.

Even if this seems like very strange stuff to you, next time you are eating chew your food thoroughly and be aware of the feeling of it rolling around your tongue. I noticed a lot of new awareness, and I look forward to continuing the practice of transferring the Prana from my foods.

The moral of the story of our mouth is that we can improve our digestion and our health, by eating less complex foods, in less complex combinations and by chewing more.

Next we'll take a look at the stomach, the place where the digestive system really gets into some serious work.

Our Stomach

I promise that I will not bore you with a complete and thorough discussion of the chemistry of the stomach. That can be found online for those wishing to understand the process in depth.

We will limit our discussion to the basics that need to be understood to make better eating choices to enable efficient and effective digestion.

After food has been well chewed and moved out of the mouth via the esophagus, it encounters gastric juices produced by the stomach which contain hydrochloric acid and two enzymes: pepsin and gastric lipase. Pepsin acts to break down protein, and lipase helps in digestion of fats but also in sterilization of the intestinal tract. The acid provides the optimal pH for the enzymes to work.

Once the food reaches the stomach, the stomach's muscle contractions begin to thoroughly mix the food with the digestive juices to stimulate the chemical breakdown of the food.

There are three key factors in our discussion of the stomach.

1. Gastric Juice Production is Limited

Number one is that gastric juices are produced in limited quantities each day. Typically there are enough to digest two large meals. Snacking on heavy foods between meals does not allow time for the body to restock the gastric juices which means that at some point in the day, the digestive system will "run out of juice" and digestion will be greatly diminished.

2. Our Stomach Needs Room to Work

Another key point is the stomach must use muscle churning to mix its digestive chemicals with the incoming food. If we eat too much, and fill our stomach beyond 80% capacity, then it is much more difficult for the stomach to mix the food and the digestive juices, which inhibits digestion.

Take a jar and add any powder to it and then fill it to the absolute top with water and put the lid on. Then slowly shake it up and down a few times to see how well the powder gets mixed with the liquid; probably not very well as there is no space to create movement.

Now try the same experiment with the jar only 80% filled with liquid and you'll understand why we must not over-fill our stomachs with food. Our stomach must have room to blend the enzymes by creating motion with the liquid food and our digestive juices.

3. Don't Mix Starches with Proteins

The third important point is that the stomach is primarily for protein digestion. When a starchy or carb food is eaten alone, the secretions in the stomach do not contain the intense acid necessary for protein digestion, therefore allowing the carbohydrate digestion to continue as the food passes into the small intestine.

When protein and starch are eaten together, the acid released in the stomach to digest the protein, stops the digestion of the carbs because the pH of the stomach kills the digestive enzymes for carbohydrate digestion that were started in the mouth. The bottom line is that when proteins and carbs are eaten together, then neither one can be properly digested.

Timing is Everything

The other very important thing we need to look at is the speed that foods leave the stomach. Water and liquids are the quickest to leave the stomach, fruits, with their high water content and low fiber take slightly longer in the stomach. Starches or carbohydrates take longer and proteins take even longer than starches. Fats are the slowest foods to exit the stomach.

Unlike the small and large intestine, our body alerts us to digestive problems in the stomach by burping and acid reflux.

Since different foods require different times in the stomach and different environments in the stomach, it is so important for us to know the guidelines of food combining and, if we are going to eat a variety of foods in the same meal, to make sure the mixture results in a harmonious journey through our digestive system, rather than a case of indigestion and gas.

Our Small Intestine

When food has been processed by the stomach it moves along into the small intestine. The small intestine is the most important part of the digestive system, since it is responsible for most of the extraction of nutrients from our food. The nutrients must be broken down into small enough particles to pass through the walls of the small intestine and into the bloodstream. From there they are carried to the rest of the body where they are employed for energy or repair work.

The small intestine continues the work of the stomach, breaking down foods into the basic components of proteins (amino acids), fats (fatty acids) and starches (sugars) which can be used by the body. It is the longest section of the digestive system, because the process needs to be slow to allow for maximum absorption of nutrients from our food.

It is in the small intestine where we first have the possibility of indigestion and gas. Gas is caused by bacteria interacting with undigested foods, usually starches. Normally this process only happens in the colon or large intestine, which contains vast amounts of bacteria, but these bacteria, can be found in the small intestine as well if undigested food is being chronically passed into the small intestine.

The formula is pretty simple, the more undigested food the bacteria have, whether in the small intestine or the colon, the more gas will be created.

When we eat a meal that is difficult to digest, we are feeding the bacteria and making them stronger, which will eventually lead to symptoms of poor health.

The small intestine is a very complex and vitally important part of our body. It is responsible for the extraction of the nutrients: amino acids, sugars and fats from our foods that give us life. It is essential to our health that it be healthy and any "mistakes" that we make in food selection, food combining and lack of chewing all put stress on and inhibit the small intestine from being able to do its job of creating a wonderful healthy body for us to use to enjoy life to its fullest.

Our Colon

The final stop on our journey through the digestive or gastrointestinal tract is our colon.

Bacterial populations in the colon or large intestine digest carbohydrates, proteins and fats that escape digestion and absorption in small intestine.

The colon is like a gas station on a deserted road.

"Last-chance Texaco."

The colon represents the last chance for the body to extract some nutrients from our food before sending the remnants to the toilet.

There are large bacterial populations in our colons and they need to be there for our health; it's not a bad thing. They are present to digest foods that were not properly digested in the small intestine.

The digestion of foods by bacteria results in fermentation and has by-products like sulfur gas, ammonia and alcohol, all of which are toxic in our body. The colon was designed to handle small bits of undigested food, which is normal as none of us eat and chew perfectly all the time.

Unfortunately, in most modern diets, even in a lot of healthy eaters, the amount of poorly digested foods entering the colon is extremely high. This results in an overgrowth of unfriendly bacteria in the colon, and even worse, massive amounts of toxic gases and other waste by products being created and released into our system.

Your Body's Text Message to You - in the Toilet

Our body gives us feedback in many ways. Symptoms of any kind are actually a form of feedback from our body to us: its "master."

Gas and indigestion are one of the milder feedback mechanisms that signal poor eating habits. The other feedback mechanism that we can use to gauge our digestive success is our stool.

Our body is incapable of lying. If something is wrong it expresses it; the only question is whether or not we will listen to the message. Take a moment to notice what comes out of your colon and plops into the toilet.

Are there bits of recognizable food in your stool? Common culprits are buckwheat, lettuce, corn, peas, or red pepper. Plain and simple, this tells us that we are not chewing enough. It is an interesting thing to notice because it really reveals to us the importance of chewing.

When a food can go 24 hours or more and remain untouched in a system that is full of chemicals and processes designed to break it down and digest it – we really begin to see how important that first step of chewing is!

The second thing to notice with undigested food, is does it have little fuzzy stuff attached to it? This is putrification, and if you have stuff like that coming out of you, you were most likely experiencing gas and indigestion as the bacteria were acting on your improperly chewed and semi-digested food. Even the bacteria couldn't finish the job!

Mucus, constipation, diarrhea, loose stools and irregular timing of bowel movements are all giving us clues about our digestive system's health. Each one of these can mean so many things that an entire book could be written about them, but what I noticed was that as I simplified my food combinations and learned to honor by body's best practices for food combining in my meals, my stools slowly improved as did my health.

Digestive System Summary

What I have presented above is an over simplification of our digestive system. There are many more organs like the liver, pancreas and gall bladder that play an important part in digestion. Also there is a lot of fantastic knowledge regarding the immune system and how its function is connected to the gastrointestinal tract. What I have done is to limit the information presented to the absolute minimum that is needed to understand food combining and to show the importance of getting aligned with the systems in our body that nourish and sustain our health.

The body tries it's best to overcome any mistakes that we make in our eating choices. But, even as magnificent as it is, it can only do so much to cope. What starts in our mouth as a yummy tasting bit of organic dried fruit from our raw granola, ends up as undigested bacteria fertilizer emitting toxic by-products into our bloodstream.

Once and a while, we can get away with a bit of gas or indigestion, but habitual poor eating choices leads our body to have to work harder and harder to extract what it needs for optimal health.

The purpose of understanding the fantastic voyage of digestion has been to illustrate the cause and effect relationship between the food choices we make and the results we experience in our body.

If we are not experiencing optimal health, then we are not putting optimal materials into our body, or as we have stressed in this book, even if we are eating high quality food, we are not putting it into our body in a way that is in alignment with the processing capabilities of our digestive system.

I'm hoping the information presented will provide you with a valuable missing piece of the puzzle to get back into a more harmonious and healthy relationship with your body.

In the next section we will tie together all of the processes and systems presented so far into some simple rules and guidelines that you can follow when you plan, prepare and eat your meals.

SECTION FOUR: GUIDELINES FOR HEALTHY FOOD COMBINING

Keeping it Simple

In this section I will outline the rules for proper food combining. Food combining is a bit like learning a language, there are simple rules and there are more complex rules and exceptions.

In my life, I've found that complexity is not my friend in most cases. The reason is that it gets overwhelming. What works for me is to start very simple and get good at the simple things before moving to the more complicated guidelines.

I've noticed that there are certain types of people that must know everything about a topic, including all the complexity, before they can take the first step. If you're one of those types of people, I urge you to try a new approach when learning food combining. Suspend your need to know more, and just take the first baby steps by implementing the simple rules as soon as possible.

The reason that this is the best approach is because food combining actually has two learning levels: the first level is the simple straightforward stuff. This is based on facts about how every human body operates. These have been discussed in this book: enzymes for different types of foods, pH levels, acid environments, digestion times etc. The simple rules of food combining are based on these proven scientific facts.

Level two is the complex stuff. The mistake people make is thinking that these more subtle "rules" are just as important as the simple rules. This is not true. They are important, but they are more about fine tuning. First we must build the foundation of proper eating and food combining and then we fine tune.

It needs to be this way because level two guidelines are personal. Level two guidelines may not be the same for everyone, and they need to be based on feedback from your body. But until you master the simple food combining rules and have re-established a healthy relationship with eating and your body, you can't trust the feedback you are receiving.

Based on what I learned from my education at the Hippocrates Health Institute, I'm going to give you the simplest and most powerful tools for understanding food combining. They are the two principles and five simple rules of food combining. Following these simple facts has made a dramatic change in the way I eat, and a corresponding improvement in my health.

Two Principles of Food Combining

There are really only two things that are important in the digestive process: each type of food requires a specific environment (pH level) with specific enzymes and gastric juices to digest it, and each food type requires different times to digest. Everything to do with food combining can be traced back to these two simple concepts.

Principle One: Maintain Pure Digestive Environments

Protein foods need an acidic digestive environment in the stomach to be properly broken down and digested.

Carbohydrate or starchy foods need the alkaline fluids that come from our saliva to be properly digested.

When acids in the stomach mix with the alkaline digestive enzymes that are used in the mouth for starch digestion, they neutralize them.

It is not possible for the body to digest protein and starch at the same time as it cannot maintain both an alkaline stomach for the starch and an acidic stomach for the protein.

Principle Two: Keep the Slow Foods out of the Fast Lane

We have all had the frustrating experience of being in a hurry and being stuck behind someone who is clueless and driving in the fast lane at exactly the same speed as the car next to them in the slow lane!

Our digestive system is just like that but even worse, as there is only a single lane on a one way street!

Different types of foods digest at different speeds. They are all like cars with only one speed. If you put a slower food in front of a faster food, frustration, in the form of fermentation is the result.

For optimal digestion food needs to move through the gastrointestinal (GI) tract at its correct speed. If it gets slowed down, the result is indigestion and toxic by-products like alcohol and gas.

Two things to remember from this principle: eat foods that take less time to digest first, so they don't get slowed down by other foods and after eating slower foods, wait a sufficient amount of time before introducing new faster digesting foods into the system.

Before we move on the rules of food combining, the next section is a quick reference guide of digestive times for all the major food types.

Digestive Times for Food Types

This section is a reference guide to help implement the "fast cars, slow cars" digestive speed guidelines presented in the previous section. Since the digestive tract is a single-lane one-way highway, to avoid upset and digestive frustration, faster-digesting foods must always be eaten before slower-digesting ones.

The following are the times that various foods spend in the stomach. Once foods get released from the stomach, they all travel through the rest of the digestive system at pretty much the same speed. For the sake of completeness, I am including foods that would never be found on a raw or vegan diet, but it helps to better understand the food categories.

Proteins

Proteins take 4 - 5 hours to digest. Nuts, seeds (and animal flesh foods including dairy).

Carbohydrates

Carbohydrates or more accurately starches, take 2 - 3 hours to digest. Examples are: grains, cooked beans, peas. Also this group includes starchy vegetables like: butternut squash, acorn squash, yams and potatoes.

Vegetables

Vegetables take 2 - 3 hours to digest. Green sprouts like sunflowers, peas and alfalfa, leafy greens, most other common vegetables and small sprouted beans like lentils.

This category also includes smoothies made from vegetables. Even though they are in liquid form, they are still just diluted whole foods, which does not really speed up digestion.

Sweet Fruits

Sweet fruits take 1/2 - 2 hours to digest. Ripe bananas (unripe ones are very hard for the body to digest and not recommended), figs and dried fruits like raisons, goji berries and dates.

Subacid Fruits

Subacid fruits take 1 1/2 to 2 hours to digest. Peaches, cherries, grapes, mangoes, pears and most other common fruits that are not citrus fruits.

Acid Fruits

Acid fruits take 1 to 1 1/2 hours to digest. Citrus fruits like grapefruit, oranges and lemons as well as strawberries and pineapple.

Melons

Melons (watermelon, cantaloupe and honeydew etc.) take 15 to 30 minutes to digest.

An easy way to remember the digestive speed of the fruits is that they are roughly ordered by their water content. Melons are almost all water so they digest, by far the fastest. Citrus and pineapple are very high in water (juice) content compared to cherries or pears, which are in turn very high in water content compared to bananas or dried fruits. More water equals less time in the stomach.

Juices

Juices take 15 minutes or less to move out of the stomach. Water goes out of the stomach almost immediately and other *fresh* vegetable and fruit juices can move out in as little as 15 minutes.

Vegetables and fruits should not be mixed in the same juice as they have different digestive environments and times.

Juices also need to be "chewed" i.e. mixed with saliva before they are swallowed to be digested properly.

Fats

Add as much as two to three hours to digestion of other foods.

A salad of leafy green vegetables will take two to three hours to digest but if a dressing that contains olive, sunflower or any other oil in any significant amount is added to the salad, the digestion time of that salad can double, which is bad news for the digestion of the green vegetables.

This is because the salad or other foods are coated in oil and the oil must be digested first, as it protects the underlying foods from digesting. By the time the oil has been processed by our digestive juices, the leafy green vegetables may have begun to ferment.

Avocados

Avocados can digest anywhere from 15 minutes to 2 hours. They should only be eaten with subacid fruits, acid fruits, and vegetables or alone.

Summary of Digestive Times

Eat foods that digest ultra quickly, like melons, alone.

From there, eat the quicker foods before any other foods if you are eating them at the same meal. Never eat foods with different digestive times in combination.

If you do eat a slow to digest food, like a protein, you must allow enough time for it to clear the stomach, up to four hours, before eating any other quick to digest foods as your stomach need to completely change its environmental conditions, its pH level, to process the new food.

There is one other piece of information about time that I'd like to share. It is not related to food combining directly but has been an important piece of the health puzzle for me.

Snacking

Our body needs time between meals to rest. During the break between meals our body replenishes the digestive juices and enzymes needed to process the next meal.

The best is to have only water, fresh juice or fruit (on an empty stomach) between meals, as heavier foods will put stress on the digestive system.

The other time when it is important not to snack is after dinner. When we sleep our body goes into a rest and repair cycle. Digestion is actually the most labor intensive process in the body, so if we still have food in our stomach when we go to bed, our energy goes to digestion rather than cellular repair or for use in the immune system.

Therefore, if most meals take three to four hours to leave the stomach, it is best if the last solid food we eat is three to four hours before we lay down for the night.

A reminder that I have prepared a printable food classification chart and summary of the food combining rules which is available here: FartFreeVegan.com/chart

Food Classifications and Combining Rules

As I mentioned previously due to the science involved, food combining can become quite complex. To me, complexity is the enemy, especially when first starting out, so I have tried to simplify everything down to its vital essence.

The next section has two parts: the first is a list of foods and their classification and the second is the rules of food combining which will draw on the food classification list.

Food Classifications List

The following is a list of foods and their classifications. Refer to it when you are learning the food combining principles and guidelines.

I've included some foods that are not found on a vegan or raw foodie's diet, because we all fall off the horse once in a while and also it helps to have a better overall understanding of food.

I have also included many foods on this list that I personally do not eat, and do not consider healthy food choices, but this is a food classification chart and not a shopping list. As you improve and learn to listen to your body, you will naturally understand which foods do not have a beneficial effect on your health.

One other thing to mention again is that foods are never 100% protein or starch. All foods have a mixture of fats, starches and proteins. The classifications below are by the dominant aspect of each food. Surprisingly, while our body has a difficult time when we mix proteins and starch foods for example, our GI system handles a food that is a mixture of protein and starch as long as it is taken into the system alone. Like many things in life: simplicity is the key.

Protein Foods

Raw Nuts: pecans, almonds, Brazil nuts, hazelnuts, walnuts, macadamias, pistachios, pine nuts, cashews.

Seeds: sunflower seeds, sesame seeds, pumpkin and squash seeds.

All nuts and seeds (as well as grains) should be soaked, at least overnight, to release enzyme inhibitors. Enzyme inhibitors are a natural form of protection that nuts and seeds (and beans) have that make them very difficult to digest. Soaking destroys the enzyme inhibitors and activates the living enzymes within the nuts, seeds and beans and turns them from being dormant, to a living food.

Low Protein: avocados (also a fat), olives, milk (not recommended).

Animal Proteins (not recommended): cheese (raw milk or unprocessed), eggs, all flesh foods except fat.

Starches (Also Called Carbs or Carbohydrates)

All starches are carbohydrates, but not all carbohydrates are starchy. For example, honey and other sugars are carbohydrates, but they are not starchy. Starches contain cellulose (fiber), and that is the real distinction between a starch and a carb. Grapes are carbohydrate, but they are not starch. Breads are both a carbohydrate and a starch as are lentils.

Starchy Proteins (Combine as starch): beans, peas, lentils, peanuts (are a legume not a nut and not recommended because they can contain funguses and toxins), chestnuts.

Grains: wild rice, rice, buckwheat, millet, wheat, rye, barley, oats and amaranth. All grains should be soaked at least overnight before eating, even if you are cooking them.

Mildly Starchy Vegetables: carrots, artichokes, beets, rutabaga, winter squash (acorn, butternut, pumpkin), water chestnuts, sprouted grains.

Starchy Vegetables: white potatoes, yams and sweet potatoes, mature corn, Jerusalem artichokes, and parsnips.

Green and Non Starchy Vegetables: spinach, Swiss chard, beet tops, rhubarb, lettuce, celery, cabbage (young, sweet), cucumber, cauliflower, sweet pepper, broccoli, Brussels sprouts, kale, collard greens, dandelion greens, okra, kohlrabi, turnips, eggplant, green young corn, green beans (young & tender), zucchini (and all other summer squash) , bok choy, alfalfa and other green sprouts, ocean vegetables and seaweeds.

Use the following vegetables in limited quantities, if at all, as they can be difficult to digest: parsley, watercress, chives, scallions, onions, leeks, radishes, garlic.

Syrups and Sugars:* brown sugar, "raw" sugar, white sugar, milk sugar, maple syrup, cane syrup, corn syrup, honey, agave.

*None of these are recommended in a healthy diet. Personally, the only sweetener that I use is stevia.

Fats

Good Fats (in small quantities): seeds, nuts, avocados, coconut meat.

Oils:* olive oil, coconut oil, sesame oil, sunflower seed oil, corn oil, peanut oil, cottonseed oil, safflower oil.

Animal Fats (not recommended): butter, cream, fats in fleshy meats.

Synthetic Fats (not recommended): margarine, Fat substitutes like olestra (Olean) found in "low fat" foods. These foods are indigestible - avoid!

*Personally I avoid oils as much as possible because they are concentrated foods. It takes 44 olives to make a tablespoon of olive oil and even if you feel like eating 44 olives, you are leaving out all the fiber and nutrients the body expects to be included. My motto is "whole foods are best."

If you do use oils, use unrefined cold-pressed certified organic oils which are less likely to be rancid.

Fruits

Acid Fruits
- **Fresh Sweet Acid Fruits**: bananas, persimmons, all sweet grapes, fresh figs.
- **Dried Acid Fruits**: dates, figs, raisins, prunes, apricots, peaches, apples, cherries, bananas, any other dried fruits.

Subacid Fruits: apples, peaches, nectarines, pears, cherries, papayas, mangos, apricots, plums, blueberries, raspberries, blackberries, cherimoyas.

Acid Fruits: oranges, grapefruit, lemons, limes, pineapples, strawberries, pomegranates, kiwi fruit, cranberries, sour acid fruits: apples, grapes, cherries.

Tomatoes are an acid fruit, without the sugar content. Use in vegetable salad or with any non-starchy vegetables, but not in a starch meal.

Melons: watermelon, honeydew melon, cantaloupe, muskmelon.

Now that we have classified all the most common foods we can use the classifications to present the simple rules for food combining.

Now that we have a classification list clearly showing the types of foods, and we have presented in the previous chapter the way the body digests each type of food, we can tie them both together with some simple rules that will align our eating to our body's digestive processes.

Five Food Combining Rules for a Happy Belly

What I present below are a simplified set of food combining rules that, if followed, will make a dramatic change in your digestive comfort level and your body awareness. Like they did for me, I hope they will improve your health and even your level of happiness.

#1 The Protein and Starch Rule

NEVER eat protein foods and starchy or carb foods at the same meal.

Either one can be eaten with non-starchy or leafy vegetables, but never have them both together.

#2 The Starches and Acid Foods Rule

NEVER combine starches or carbs with acid foods.

Acid foods are the proteins, but also: coffee and teas, honey, cocoa, mustard, vinegar and alcohol. Also all the most common fruits are acid fruits. Coconut, rice and soy milks are also mildly acid and should not be mixed with starchy foods like grains, rice, sprouted beans or legumes or starchy vegetables.

#3 The Fruit Rules

(Four little rules to make one rule!)

Best to eat fruits on an empty stomach.

ALWAYS eat melons alone.

NEVER combine fruits with foods that have a longer digestive time like starches or proteins. If you must eat them both at the same meal, separate them and eat the fruits first, then wait 20 minutes or longer before eating the protein or starch.

Fruits (except melons) are okay with raw greens.

#4 The Fatty Food Rule

Eat fatty foods VERY sparingly and eat them alone if possible.

Vegan fatty foods include avocados, nuts and seeds and oils. All fatty foods delay digestion and therefore create problems when mixed with other foods that need to digest more quickly. Oils are the worst as they are a concentrated food, so they are the most harmful when mixed with other foods.

If you are going to eat nuts, seeds or avocado with other foods, eat them at the end of your meal to minimize delays to the rest of the food you have eaten.

#5 The Vegetable Rule

Vegetables (non starchy) are great with starches and they are great with proteins. Just don't have starches and proteins at the same meal.

5 Most Common Food Combination Mistakes

Mistake #1 Fruits

Eating fruit with grains, starches or nuts.

This one is going to be a shock for some vegans and raw foodies, but if you do it, it hurts your gut. This rule calls into question most desserts and granolas and a lot of smoothies.

I'm not saying that you should never do it, because we all need a little fun, but if you're having digestive problems on an otherwise healthy vegan diet, the way you're using fruit is the first place to look.

Fruit digests more quickly than other foods, and it will begin to ferment if it is mixed with slower digesting foods and that will cause bloating and gas due to unhealthy bacterial activity.

If you must eat fruit with anything other than green veggies, eat it on an empty stomach and wait at least 20 minutes before eating anything else.

Mistake #2 Smoothies

Overly complicated green smoothies.

Smoothies are the fast food of the raw and vegan diet lifestyle. Green smoothies can be like health food garbage cans, with people believing the more things that come from the health food store that they blend up into a smoothie, the healthier they are going to get.

Keep green smoothies simple! The best is just green veggies. From there you can try some fruits - but pay attention to your body, if you get gas then the smoothie is too complex. Never use packaged or bottled fruit juices, syrup or sugar or dates in your smoothie. These foods are too condensed. If you have to sweeten your smoothie, use a bit of stevia or a banana as a last resort.

Mistake #3 Avocados

Avocados with nuts or tomatoes.

The fat in avocados slows down digestion of any foods they are eaten with. This is bad news for the proteins in nuts or seeds, and especially with tomatoes which are a fast digesting fruit.

Avocados in your smoothie? Only if it doesn't have nuts or seeds (or nut or seed milk). If it just has green veggies then you're fine.

No guacamole?

If you're like me you're thinking, "oh my god!" what about guacamole? Don't worry, substitute red pepper for the tomatoes.

You'll be surprised the Aztecs didn't use peppers when they invented it, guacamole is way better with peppers replacing the tomatoes!

And in my house we use cucumbers as dippers to replace the corn chips, or put the guacamole in a Nori wrap (the seaweed used to make sushi) with salad and you'll have an amazingly yummy wrap.

Mistake #4 Nuts and Oils

Nuts with olive or any other oil.

Similar to avocados with nuts, olive oil is a fat, and a condensed food which is even more intense to digest than an avocado.

The oil will slow down digestion when mixed with nuts. This calls into question quite a few raw and vegan salad dressings and sauces like pesto that use oils as a thickener and nuts or nut milks to make them creamy.

Try a pinch of xanthan gum to get that thick sensation in salad dressings so you don't miss the oil. As for pesto, the most authentic and original Italian pesto doesn't have pine nuts in it. Just leave the nuts out, or substitute a bit of zucchini if you still want a bulky texture to your pesto.

Mistake #5 Nut Milks and Grains

Using nut milks with grains.

Hemp milk or almond milk on top of any type of cereal; buckwheat, quinoa, millet etc, will cause digestive problems.

The first commandment of food combining is to never mix proteins and starches. They require completely different types of enzymes and different digestive environments in the stomach to properly digest. If you eat them together, you force the body into a no win situation in which neither one gets properly digested properly.

I do love having a liquid on my cereals, luckily there are some solutions. You can make milk from quinoa or buckwheat and then use it on your cereal. Add a tiny bit of xanthan gum as a thickener and a bit of vanilla bean and a bit of stevia.

The other thing that can work is to make milk from Sunwarrior Powder (see resources). Technically it is called "protein powder" but it is made from brown rice, so I find that I can use it with starchy foods. I recommend conducting your own experiment. Use it on your cereal, make sure you chew your meal really well, and then if you don't have any indigestion, it probably means that the combination works for you.

Caveats: of course there shouldn't be any fruit, dried or fresh, mixed with a food that is starchy like grains, and any grains should always be sprouted before being eaten, even if they are cooked.

Summary of the Five Mistakes

By just removing these five raw foodie and vegan food combining mistakes, you will experience a huge difference in your eating and digesting experiences. When you are eating this diet for health reasons, and not experiencing the results that you were expecting, the first place to start is by examining the food combinations.

Most raw and vegan recipes are created to taste great, unfortunately at the expense of being in harmony with our digestive system. With greater awareness we can create meals that taste great and will allow our body to benefit from the wholesome foods that we are eating.

SECTION FIVE: FINAL THOUGHTS

The reason I wrote this book was because I saw so many friends and people I met struggling with a raw or vegan diet. They were sincerely making an effort to follow what should be a very healthy way of eating, yet they were complaining of constant indigestion, low energy and lack of improvement in their health and ultimately giving up on a diet that I know does work.

Without knowledge and practice of the rules of food combining, even eating the best foods can result in our body's inability to digest causing fermentation, putrification, gas and ultimately a toxic nightmare in our digestive system that leads to disease.

Along the way we experience low energy, and dwindling health as the nutrients in our food are wasted and turned into food for unhealthy gut bacteria that lead to premature aging, stress and weight gain.

With what I learned while at the Hippocrates Health Institute, I knew the problem had a simple solution that involved common, yet somehow secret wisdom.

Staying healthy and feeling good is not hard. But the constant battles that most of us have with our health and maintaining a positive feeling about ourselves continue even though we are "doing all the right things" that should make us healthy.

I believe that food combining is the golden thread that will tie all the other healthy efforts together. If you follow these simple rules and align your eating with a respect for the limitations and needs of your body, then you will start to find the effortless health and progress that you have been seeking.

If it wasn't for the rules of food combining and my raw vegan diet, I would not be sitting here today writing this book.

Emotional Eating

Another important factor in my recovery from illness was to realize that a lot of my eating had more to do with trying to make myself feel better emotionally rather than nourishing my body.

It may seem strange, but eating can definitely be an addiction, especially eating certain types of fatty, high-carb and sweet foods that we know are not good for us.

Food addiction is a topic for another book entirely, but I mention it to help raise your awareness about why you might be having trouble reaching your health goals.

Eating can be a form of self love, or self loathing. Once I became aware of this fact, it was really clear to me which one I was doing when I ate.

It has been my experience that there is no way to *discipline* yourself to stop eating unhealthy foods. Willpower will not work. The only thing that worked for me was to do spend more time reinforcing the self love.

If I ate something that was "bad" for me, rather than beat myself up, I simply learned to refocus on what I wanted, which was perfect health, and to then immediately take a step in that direction, which usually meant making a green juice.

I would eat two or three chocolate bars and then drink an amazing fresh green juice 15 minutes later. It was totally disgusting, but I was training myself to be in control of my eating, to consciously choose to be healthy, and over time, the cravings for the chocolate bars diminished and the love of the healthy foods grew.

The other way to combat emotional eating is to stop and ask yourself what you are feeling as you reach for that food that you don't really want to eat. For me there was always something going on under the surface: anxiety, fear, anger or loneliness that was causing me to use food to try and numb my uncomfortable feeling.

What can work in that circumstance is to tell yourself that it's okay to feel sad, or depressed, or lonely. It isn't really the feeling that causes us to be upset, it's the inability to accept the feeling as a normal part of life that creates tension and pain inside of us. All feelings are okay, they are just feelings, and they will dry up like a puddle on a hot sunny day if we will acknowledge them and release them.

Body Awareness

This book has presented some rules that if followed will produce great results on the road to health.

However, the real goal of life, in my opinion, is not just to follow some set of external rules, but to gain awareness. Slowing down and chewing a lot will help grow this connection. Feel the food on your tongue, feel it begin to liquefy as you chew it more and more.

Enjoy the sensation of swallowing and pushing the foods down into your stomach and turning them over to and the rest of your digestive tract.

Pay attention after your meal for feedback from your digestive system. Did you overeat or was there a feeling that your stomach had enough room to mix the contents for proper enzyme reaction?

Check in with your body an hour after you eat, how is everything sitting now? And then 24 to 36 hours later, when the stool from this well combined and properly chewed meal is released into your toilet, what do you see? Any small pieces that could be chewed better? Any differences in consistency from your previous stool patterns?

How is your energy level after a light and well combined meal? Have patience for improvements, changing your diet is not a quick fix to perfect health. Sometimes there is a transition time that is required. Look for small signs of improvement, and use these as motivation to keep going forward to get to the big and fantastic improvements.

When I first stopped eating my beloved bed time snacks, I woke up feeling a lack of energy during my morning workouts. Eventually my body adjusted to the changes and I began to feel better than ever, but it can take time for real changes to show up, so don't be discouraged, if it takes a while for your lifelong bad habits to diminish as you normalize. Celebrate the small victories along the way that let you know you are on the right track.

Putting it into Practice

There is a wise saying that applies to making the changes required to become a conscious food combiner:

"How do you eat an elephant?"

"One bite at a time!"

Now, I don't recommend eating an elephant, or any other meat for that matter! But the point is that making change is a process of doing small changes, consistently over time.

If you are used to eating all the foods in the "Common Mistakes" section, focus on one mistake at a time and try to correct it.

Make one meal a week, a meal of proper food combining. And then tell yourself, "Great job, you made a step forward today!"

When I first came back from Hippocrates Health Institute, I had eaten a perfect diet for three weeks while I was there but I came home to a life that was at complete odds to everything I had learned. Even though I was highly motivated and desperate due to my illness, it took me six weeks to fully transition to my new diet.

Trying to make a big change all at once is the path to failure for most people. Make one positive step and then another tiny positive step. Eventually you'll be in love with taking the positive steps and you'll be unstoppable.

We don't need to be perfect, and we never will be! You will, like I did and still do, occasionally fall down. The only thing that matters is to get back up and keep going towards where you want to be!

I sincerely hope that this book will help you on your journey to perfect health and a fantastic experience with your own body.

Please feel free to get in touch with me at my website: JonSymons.com or on Facebook: Facebook.com/jonsymons or email me at jon@jonsymons.com

Also, if you liked this book, I'd really appreciate it if you would leave a review on Amazon by going here: FartFreeVegan.com/amazon. That will really help spread the word about food combining and hopefully make small difference in the health of many people.

If you missed it at the beginning make sure you grab a printable copy of the food combining chart and rules, so you have it for quick reference: FartFreeVegan.com/chart.

Recommended Resources

My Favorite Products

During the course of this book I realize that I have mentioned a few products and tools that I have discovered and used as a raw foodie.

So I thought I would compile a list and to share them with you and save you time and trial and error trying to find things that work and are great quality.

Simple stuff like "raw" and non-chemical digestive enzymes, to my favorite juicer to the most amazing raw vanilla powder that is incredibly affordable and 100 times better tasting than vanilla extract.

I've put the list on my website FartFreeVegan.com/I-use

Recommended Books

Vegan Diet

The China Study: The Most Comprehensive Study of Nutrition Ever Conducted

Eat to Live: The Amazing Nutrient-Rich Program for Fast and Sustained Weight Loss, Revised Edition

Forks Over Knives - The Cookbook: Over 300 Recipes for Plant-Based Eating All Through the Year

Food Combining

Clean Gut: The Breakthrough Plan for Eliminating the Root Cause of Disease and Revolutionizing Your Health

VB6: Eat Vegan Before 6:00 to Lose Weight and Restore Your Health . . . for Good

Food Combining & Digestion: 101 Ways to Improve Digestion

Food Combining: 4 Page Bi-Fold Laminated Reference Cards - Learn Tips, Tricks & Recipes For Raw & Living Food Diet Food Combinations (Permacharts: Raw Foods Vegetarianism)

Fit for Life A classic that introduced me to food combining many years ago.

Credits

I am deeply grateful to Brian and Anna Maria Clement for their lifetime commitment to helping people understand how the human body works and providing people with the tools to heal using a living foods raw vegan diet. You can find more information about what they do on their website: http://www.hippocratesinst.org/

I am grateful to the following websites for sharing their knowledge online.

http://www.stylenectar.com/stylenectar/2013/03/proper-food-combining-the-missing-cornerstone-to-a-healthy-beautiful-body-anti-aging-energy.html

http://www.rawfoodexplained.com/science.html

http://thechalkboardmag.com/food-combining-6-common-raw-food-combos-that-wreak-havoc-on-your-health

COPYRIGHT NOTICE

Made in the USA
Lexington, KY
09 October 2014